Crock-pot Recipes

60 Easy, Delicious, and Healthy Crock-pot Recipes for Busy People

Table of Contents

Introduction

Congratulations on purchasing your personal copy of *Crock-pot Recipes: 60 Easy, Delicious, and Healthy Crock-pot Recipes for Busy People.* Thank you for doing so.

It's incredible that Crock-pots are not more common because there are countless benefits to doing so, and not so many disadvantages. These wonderful machines have existed since your grandma's day and were used a lot back then, for good reason. Actually, that's how our grandmas and moms made such great home cooked meals while still having time to go to work or take care of the house! You can use your Crock-pot multiple times every week. For those who work from home, a Crock-pot helps you stay on task with your work, while those who have to leave the house to work can also benefit from one.

7 Reasons to Use your Crock-pot more often:

Still not convinced? Let's look at the benefits to using your Crock-pot instead of cooking at home or going to a restaurant.

Reason 1: They save you Energy.

A Crock-pot doesn't take up as much electricity as using an oven. If you're the type who uses electricity for cooking, a Crock-pot will save you money on your power bill.

Reason 2: It always you to Multitask.

Any time you use your Crock-pot, you are able to take care of other things as your meal is cooking. Perhaps the greatest advantage of a Crock-pot over more traditional cooking methods is that you don't have to stir or watch your food as it cooks! Actually, it's usually recommended not to open the lid as soon as you've begun cooking because this can slow it down.

Reason 3: It Saves you Money.

With a Crock-pot, you can now purchase those less-than-perfect cuts of meat. Although cooking them in the oven or on the stove would usually result in a tough consistency, your slow cooking Crock-pot will soften them up until they're nice and tender.

Reason 4: Your Food doesn't Burn as Easily.

Not everyone is blessed with the ability to make food perfectly every time, and even those who don't always want the hassle of hovering over the stove all day. With a Crock-pot, you are far less likely to burn or scorch your food since the machine uses low temperatures.

Reason 5: Your Stovetop will be Free.

When you use a Crock-pot, your stovetop and oven will be free for other tasks that otherwise wouldn't be possible. During the holiday season, this is especially helpful. Now you can make many dishes at once using your oven, stove, and Crock-pot.

Reason 6: They don't Create Extra Heat.

The stovetop heats your kitchen up, which is nice in some seasons, but not so nice in the summer. With a Crock-pot, you can make your favorite dishes without worrying about the discomfort of extra heat in your kitchen during the warm seasons.

Reason 7: Your Meals are Healthier.

Typically, meals made in the Crock-pot have less fat in them because the foods are allowed to cook without any extra oil or butter. The meats included simmer in their own natural juices.

These are only seven of the countless reasons why using your Crock-pot is a great idea. If you aren't taking advantage of this wonderful machine, you're missing out! Not only is it more convenient, but the food that comes out of a Crock-pot has, even more, flavor than stovetop dishes, which may end up too cooked. If you're ready to learn more about what your Crock-pot can do, keep reading.

There are plenty of books on this subject on the market, thanks again for choosing this one! Every effort was made to ensure it is full of as much useful information as possible. Please enjoy!

Chapter 1
Easy Slow Cooked Meals

A well-balanced diet full of nutrients, in addition to regular exercise and avoiding bad habits like smoking, is what it takes to reach optimal health. Healthy eating means ingesting plenty of quality proteins, fats that are healthy for the heart, minerals, good carbohydrates, water, and vitamins in the dishes you eat. You should also minimize saturated fats, processed food sources, and drinking alcohol. Sticking to a diet like this will allow you to keep a healthy body weight, perform your daily functions with ease and comfort, and keep away harmful diseases. Without further ado, let's get to some recipes that fit into this mold, so you can stay healthy!

Recipe #1: Flavorful Chili.

This is a classic, but always a favorite, especially in the cold winter months!

Ingredients you need:

- A pound of ground meat, drained and cooked.

- One big yellow or white onion.

- Three cans of kidney beans, strained.

- Two cans of chopped tomatoes.

- Tomato sauce (one large can).

- Three tablespoons of chili powder.

- Pepper and salt (as you prefer).

- Hot sauce (if you want it).

Instructions to make:

1. This recipe is very simple. Just throw all of these ingredients into the Crock-pot and let it cook on low heat for up to eight hours. You can add more seasonings once it's done depending on your preference.

Recipe #2: Chicken Tortilla Stew.

Ingredients you need:

- One pound of chicken fillets (boneless).

- One can of chopped tomatoes.

- Half a cup of salsa (chunky).

- One cup of enchilada sauce.

- One can of strained black beans.

- One large white onion, diced.

- A few cloves of chopped garlic.

- Four cups of chicken broth.

- Two teaspoons of cumin.

- One teaspoon of chili powder.

- One teaspoon of lemon juice.

Instructions to make:

1. Put your Crock-pot on high, then add the chicken into the pot (chopped) along with the broth and diced onion, then stir gently. Or you can add the entire filets of chicken and shred them up one they have cooked.

2. Add the rest of the ingredients on the list and put your Crock-pot onto a lower heat setting, letting it cook for a few hours.

3. Serve with avocado, cilantro, and sour cream if desired.

Recipe #3: Creamy Pork Loin.

One of the fancier meals on our list, this dish has a creamy filling of goat cheese, lemony herbs, and silky spinach, making it healthy and delicious. The dish has apricot-flavored sauce. To make the meat even nicer, you can brown it in a pan before you place it into your Crock-pot. You can serve this meal with green beans and mashed potatoes or with garlic-flavored Brussel sprouts.

Ingredients you need:

- Two separate tablespoons of fresh olive oil.

- Half a cup of shallots (sliced thinly).

- One tablespoon of diced garlic.

- One small package of spinach.

- Three ounces of fresh goat cheese.

- Two tablespoons of chives (fresh).

- Two tablespoons of fresh parsley.

- One teaspoon of lemon peel (ground).

- Three pounds of pork loin (boneless).

- One tablespoon of fresh thyme (chopped).

- Two tablespoons of butter (unsalted).

- One tablespoon of mustard (Dijon).

- Two tablespoons of vinegar.

- Salt and pepper to taste.

- A quarter cup of apricot preserves.

Instructions to make:

1. Heat up the olive oil in a large pan over medium heat, then add the thyme, garlic, and shallots, stirring often until the shallots are browned. Add your spinach to the mix and let it cook lightly with constant stirring until the leaves have wilted, then take them off the heat.

2. Mix the lemon rind, parsley, chives, and goat cheese into a bowl.

3. Cut your meat horizontally without piercing through the other side of it, then open the meat up. Beginning at the middle, cut again through both halves of meat horizontally, without piercing through to the other size. On both sides, open flat, then put the pork between plastic wrap (two sheets).

4. Pound the meat until it's all half an inch thick using a skillet or meat mallet, then take the plastic wrap off.

5. Season the meat with salt and pepper to your liking, then mix the cheese blend over the meat evenly. Top this with the mixture of shallots and roll it together like jelly rolls. This can be tied using cooking twine every inch or so, then sprinkled with some more salt and pepper.

6. Clean your pan, then heat up some more oil in your pan, adding the meat and cooking until it's browned on each side. Your pork is now ready to go into the Crock-pot.

7. Combine the mustard, butter, and apricot preserves to the pan, cooking it over medium heat for a minute until the butter has melted. Pour this mixture over the meat in the Crock-pot, setting it to low and letting it cook for up to eight hours. You will know it's done when a meat thermometer reads 145 degrees F.

8. When it's finished, put the meat onto a cutting board and let it sit for 10 minutes to cool. Discard the fat from the Crock-pot, then add sauce to a saucepan. Boil the sauce over medium heat, cooking for five minutes and reducing it to a single cup of sauce. Add the vinegar now, then throw away the twin, cut the meat, and serve it with your apricot sauce.

Recipe #4: Tasty Chicken and Vegetables.

Ingredients you need:

- Three cups of chopped carrots.

- One pound of potatoes (yellow) cut into wedges.

- Two pounds of chicken meat, boneless.

- One can of chicken broth (low sodium).

- A third of a cup of white wine (dry).

- Four garlic cloves, chopped.

- Three-quarters teaspoon of salt.

- One large can of rinsed artichoke hearts.

- Two egg yolks and one whole egg.

- A third of a cup of lemon juice.

- A third a cup of fresh dill, chopped.

- Salt and pepper.

Instructions to make:

1. Spread the potatoes and carrots over the base of your Crock-pot, then add the chicken to the top of them. Simmer your salt, garlic, wine, and broth in a saucepan over medium heat, then pour it over the veggies and chicken.

2. Cover the mixture and allow it to cook for a few hours, or until the vegetables and meat are tender. Add in your artichokes, then cover again and cook for five minutes. Whisk your lemon juice, egg yolks, and egg in a medium-sized bowl in the meantime.

3. Move the vegetables and chicken to a large serving pan with a spoon, then cover them so they stay hot. Transfer half a cup of cooking juices to the mixture of eggs and lemon juice. Cover this and cook, stirring it a few times until it gets thick. This should take about 20 minutes. Add the pepper and dill, then pour your sauce over the veggies and chicken.

Recipe #5: Pot Roast Braised in Coffee.

Ingredients you need:

- A quarter pound beef roast, fat trimmed off.

- Salt and pepper to personal taste.

- Four teaspoons of divided olive oil.

- Four chopped garlic cloves.

- One teaspoon of thyme (dried).

- One three-quarters cup of strong coffee.

- Two tablespoons apple cider vinegar.

- Two tablespoons of water mixed with cornstarch.

- Two big white onions, cut into small pieces.

Instructions to make:

1. Add the beef, seasoned with salt and pepper, to the Crock-pot, then add two teaspoons of olive oil and onions, putting the heat to medium and letting sit for 20 minutes. Add the thyme and garlic, then stir in the vinegar and coffee. Allow this to cook on low heat for a few hours or until the meat is tender.

2. When the meat is cooked, skim the fat off the top and ladle the juice from the meat into a bowl, adding the mixture of water and cornstarch to it, then whisk to create a gravy. Serve the meat with the gravy.

Recipe #6: Chicken with Tomato and Wine Braise.

For this dish, the chicken will cook in a simple, yet tasty, wine and tomato sauce. Using chicken with the bone still in will add to the heartiness of the flavor and the dish is very healthy due to using skinless meat. The extra sauce in this dish makes it perfect with brown rice and steamed broccoli on the side.

Ingredients you need:

- Four slices of bacon.

- Four garlic cloves, chopped.

- One big white onion sliced thinly.

- One teaspoon of fennel.

- One teaspoon of thyme.

- One-quarter cup of fresh parsley.

- One bay leaf.

- One can of chopped tomatoes.

- One cup of white wine (dry).

- Salt and pepper to taste.

- Four pounds of chicken thighs without skin.

Instructions to make:

1. Prepare the bacon by cooking it in a cooking pan until it's crispy, then transfer them to a paper towel to remove oil. Once they have cooled down, crumble the bacon.

2. Pour the fat from the pan but leave about two tablespoons behind to cook the onions in. Stir them until soft, then add the garlic and herbs, stirring for a couple minutes.

3. Add the white wine, allowing it to boil the mixture for two minutes and make sure you scrape up any pieces that have browned. Add in the tomatoes with the salt and tomato juice, stirring thoroughly.

4. Add the chicken thighs to your Crock-pot, then add the bacon on top of this. Next, pour your tomato sauce over the top of everything and allow it all to cook for up to six hours. When finished, take the bay leaf out and serve the dish with parsley on top.

Recipe #7: Spicy Ethiopian Chicken Stew.

This stew has been generously prepared with berbere, a famous Ethiopian spice mix. It comes with lentils and tomato and can be a spicy dish. If you don't want it too spicy, use only three spoons of spice instead of the five listed here.

Ingredients you need:

- A cup and a half of red lentils.

- Two pounds of chicken, boneless.

- Two teaspoons of olive oil.

- One tablespoon of butter.

- Four cups of red onion (diced).

- Five chopped garlic cloves.

- Half a cup of red wine (dry).

- Five tablespoons of berbere.

- One tablespoon of ginger, minced.

Instructions to make:

1. Wash the red lentils using cold water, then spread them over the bottom of your Crock-pot after draining the water. Place the pieces of chicken over this.

2. Warm up the oil and butter in a big pan over medium heat. Once this has melted completely, add the chopped onion and

stir often until cooked soft. This should require no more than six minutes. Next, add the ginger and garlic, cooking for two minutes.

3. Add the berbere spice mix and cook in the pan, then stir in the wine. Make sure you scrape the mix of onion from the pan's bottom, then add the tomatoes and juice to the mix. Add this mixture of onions to your Crock-pot, then add the broth.

4. Cover the food for up to six hours until the chicken is very tender, then mix it up so that it's all blended. Salt and pepper to taste.

Recipe #8: Swedish Ham and Pea Soup.

This soup has fresh ginger added which gives it a fuller flavor. You should use the best type of ham possible in order to add to this dish's flavor.

Ingredients you need:

- Three cups of yellow peas (split).

- Four cups of chicken broth.

- Four cups of fresh water.

- One cup of chopped carrot.

- One cup of chopped celery.

- Two cups of chopped onion (yellow).

- Eight ounces of diced ham.

- One tablespoon of fresh, chopped ginger.

- One teaspoon of marjoram (dried).

- Salt and pepper to taste.

Instructions to make:

1. Put the peas into a medium sized mixing bowl and rinse with water, then spread the drained peas into the bottom of your Crock-pot.

2. Add the water, broth, celery, carrot, onion, marjoram, ginger, and ham to your Crock-pot and stir the mixture until thoroughly blended and combined. Cover the Crock-pot and allow it to cook for six hours. This can be seasoned with salt and pepper as desired.

Recipe #9: Broth and Lamb Middle Eastern Stew.

This stew has been flavored in a bold way with typical spices from the Middle East and comes with healthy chickpeas and fresh spinach. Lamb's shoulder is both affordable and wonderfully tender when served from a Crock-pot. If you are unable to find any shoulder lamb meat without bones, just buy the shoulder cuts and take the bones out yourself. You can serve this dish with a side salad and bulgur.

Ingredients you need:

- One and a quarter pounds of lamb meat (boneless shoulder cut).

- One tablespoon of canola or olive oil (ideally olive).

- One tablespoon of coriander (ground).

- Four teaspoons of cumin (ground).

- A quarter teaspoon of cayenne pepper.

- Two medium chopped onions.

- One can of chopped tomatoes.

- One cup of chicken broth.

- Four minced garlic cloves.

- One can of rinsed chickpeas.

- Six ounces of spinach.

- Salt and pepper to taste.

Instructions to make:

1. Put the lamb meat into your Crock-pot, then mix the cumin, oil, cayenne, coriander, pepper, and salt into a small bowl on the side. Use this spice paste to coat the meat, tossing until it's completely covered. Place the onion on top.

2. Bring the garlic, broth, and tomatoes to a low boil in a saucepan, simmering lightly, then add this over the onion and lamb. Put the lid on the Crock-pot and allow it to cook for about four hours, or until the meat is tender.

3. Blot or skim any fat you see on the stew's surface. Meanwhile, mash up half a cup of chickpeas in a bowl, using a form. Mix the whole and mashed chickpeas into the Crock-pot, then add the spinach. Put the lid on and cook this, allowing the spinach to wilt, which should require only five minutes. Your dish is done!

Recipe #10: Crock-pot Bean Stew and Dumplings.

This Crock-pot dish is healthy and full of vegetables, including corn, celery, bell pepper, and onion. It's topped with crunchy chili and radish at the end and served with cornbread dumplings. You can skip the cornbread dumplings if you're short on time and instead use a bit of extra cheese and tortilla chips on top. To get the best result for your beans, soak them ahead of time so they cook all the way through in the Crock-pot.

Ingredients you need:

- One pound of dry, pre-soaked pinto beans.

- Six cups of fresh water.

- One large chopped onion.

- One diced red bell pepper.

- Two sliced celery stalks.

- One cup of canned corn.

- Two minced garlic cloves.

- Two tablespoons of powdered chili.

- Two tablespoons of fresh lime juice.

- Two teaspoons of powdered cumin.

- Half a cup of flour.

- Half a cup of cornmeal.

- Half a teaspoon of baking powder.

- Half a teaspoon of salt.

- Two tablespoons of butter (cold and cubed).

- One finely chopped fresh jalapeno.

- Lime zest.

- Half a cup of buttermilk.

- Half a cup of cilantro.

- Half a cup of sliced radishes.

Instructions to make:

1. Drain your soaked pinto beans, then mix them with the cumin, chili powder, garlic, corn, celery, bell pepper, onion, and water into your Crock-pot. Set the temperature on high for four hours.

2. In order to make the dumplings, start whisking the flour, salt, baking powder, and cornmeal just before the four hours is up. Use a pastry mixer to add the butter. Alternatively, you can use a fork to blend the butter with the dry ingredients. The end result should look like coarse meal. Add the lime zest and jalapeno, stirring thoroughly, then add the buttermilk to create a dough-like consistency.

3. Once your stew has been cooking for four hours, mix the salt and lime juice in. Spoon the dough onto the stew using generous heaps of dough, and let it sit on top. Put the lid on your Crock-pot and cook it for an hour on high. Each portion of this dish should be served with a dumpling. You may garnish it with radish and cilantro.

Chapter 2
Stay Healthy with your Crock-pot

The vitamins and nutrients present in what you eat can support your daily goals, repair damage to your cells, and protect your body from damage from your environment. Protein helps to restore injuries and adds to the health of your immune system. Fats and carbohydrates both give you the fuel you need to function, while minerals and vitamins act to support all of the processes of your body. Vitamins E, C, and A, for instance, are antioxidants that help to protect your body against toxins, while B vitamins allow you to extract useful energy from food.

Phosphorus and calcium help to strengthen your bones, while potassium and sodium help your nerve signals transmit effectively. If you don't have a healthy diet, this is all compromised. Let's look at some more ways to make sure you're getting your essential nutrients with delicious Crock-pot recipes.

Recipe #11: Crock-pot Oatmeal.

Ingredients you need:

- Eight cups of water.

- Two cups of oats (steel-cut).

- Half a cup of cranberries.

- Half a cup of dried apricots.

- Salt.

Instructions to make:

1. Mix together the apricots, cranberries, oats, water, and salt into your Crock-pot, turning it on low heat. Cover and cook, allowing the oats to get tender. This should take about eight hours.

Recipe #12: Sweet Potato and Chicken Stew.

Ingredients you need:

- Six chicken thighs with bones and the skin removed.

- Two pounds of peeled, cut sweet potatoes.

- Half a pound of white mushrooms, sliced thinly.

- Six shallots (large).

- Four peeled garlic cloves.

- Salt and pepper to taste.

- Two tablespoons of apple cider vinegar.

Instructions to make:

1. To make this dish, put the sweet potatoes, chicken, shallots, mushrooms, rosemary, wine, garlic, pepper and salt into your Crock-pot, mixing them together.

2. Cover and cook on a low heat, or until the potatoes can be pierced easily with a fork, this should require about five hours.

3. Before you serve this dish, take the bones out of the chicken and add vinegar, if desired. This can be kept in the fridge for three days or frozen for 30.

Recipe #13: Mushroom and Black Bean Chili.

Ingredients you need:

- One tablespoon of olive oil.

- One pound of black beans (dried and rinsed).

- A quarter cup of mustard seed.

- Two tablespoons of powdered chili.

- One teaspoon of ground cumin.

- Half a teaspoon of ground cardamom.

- One large white onion roughly chopped.

- One pound of sliced mushrooms.

- One small can of chopped tomatillos.

- A quarter cup of fresh water.

- 5 cups of vegetable or mushrooms broth.

- One small can of tomato paste.

- Two tablespoons of canned chipotle peppers (minced).

- A cup and a half of shredded pepper Jack cheese.

- Half a cup of sour cream (low-fat).

- Half a cup of cilantro, chopped and fresh.

- Two sliced up limes.

Instructions to make:

1. To make this recipe, soak the black beans in two-quarters of water overnight. You can also soak them by boiling them for a couple minutes and allowing them to sit for an hour. Drain the black beans and throw the soaking liquid out.

2. Mix the cardamom, cumin, chili powder, mustard seed, and oil in your Crock-pot. Turn the heat on high and stir the contents until the ingredients are sizzling, then add the water, tomatillos, mushrooms, and onions.

3. Put the lid on and cook this, while stirring it every once in a while. The vegetables should get juicy within an hour. Add the beans and allow this to cook for eight hours. Serve with some sour cream, cheese, and cilantro if desired and have lime wedges on the side.

Recipe #14: Crock-pot Chicken and Stout Stew.

Ingredients you need:

- Half a cup of flour.

- Six tablespoons of flour, separate.

- One teaspoon of salt, or however much you prefer.

- Half a teaspoon of pepper, or more if you prefer.

- Two and a half pounds of skinless, boneless chicken.

- Four teaspoons of olive oil, separated.

- Three bacon pieces, chopped up.

- One and a half cups of stout beer.

- One pound of baby carrots.

- One small package of white mushrooms, sliced.

- Two cups of onion, chopped.

- Four minced garlic cloves.

- One and a half teaspoons of thyme.

- One cup of chicken broth.

- Two cups of thawed baby peas.

Instructions to make:

1. To make this recipe, mix together six tablespoons of flour with the salt and pepper in a mixing bowl. Coat the chicken pieces in this mixture, then move them over to a nearby plate.

2. Heat up two teaspoons of olive oil in a big pan using medium heat, then add 50 percent of your chicken, cooking until it's browned (this should take about four minutes for either side). Next, transfer this meat to your Crock-pot, reducing the heat to medium. Repeat these steps with the rest of the olive oil and chicken.

3. Place the chicken into the Crock-pot and try to layer it evenly inside. Cook your bacon for two minutes, stirring frequently, then sprinkle the remaining half cup of flour over it while cooking. Add the stout beer, using a wooden spatula to get the browned pieces off the pan's bottom.

4. Pour this blend onto your meat, then add the thyme, garlic, onion, and mushrooms. Try to spread each of these over the meat evenly, then pour the broth last. This should be covered and cooked until the meat is very tender. This should require eight hours on a low heat setting or four hours on high heat.

5. The last step is to stir the peas into the mix, letting them heat all the way through. This should only take another 10 minutes. The final product can be seasoned with as much salt and pepper as you desire.

Recipe #15: Beef Goulash from Hungary.

Ingredients you need:

- Two pounds of beef chuck, cubed and trimmed.

- Two teaspoons of caraway.

- Two tablespoons of hot or sweet paprika (Hungarian).

- Salt and pepper to taste.

- Two medium sized chopped onions.

- One medium red chopped bell pepper.

- One can of chopped tomatoes.

- One can of beef broth (reduced sodium).

- One teaspoon of Worcestershire.

- Two minced garlic cloves.

- One bay leaf (or more, to taste).

- One tablespoon of cornstarch blended with water.

- Two tablespoons of fresh, chopped parsley sprigs.

Instructions to make:

1. Put the meat into a Crock-pot, then place the caraway into a small bowl, crushing if necessary. Add salt, pepper, and paprika to the mix, then sprinkle the meat with the spice

blend and make sure it's coated well. This should be topped with bell pepper and onion.

2. Blend together the Worcestershire sauce, garlic, broth, and tomatoes in a medium sized pan, simmering them over medium heat, then add the vegetables and beef. Put the bay leaf (or leaves) over the top and put the lid on.

3. Allow this mixture to cook until the meat is soft, which should take seven hours on a low heat and four hours on a high heat. Throw out the bay leaves, blot or skim any fat that is on the surface.

4. Lastly, add the mixture of cornstarch and water to the pot, cooking on a high heat and stirring a few times. This will thicken up the stew and it should be ready to serve in 15 minutes. Add parsley at the end.

Recipe #16: Crock-pot Braised Beef with Turnips and Carrots.

Ingredients you need:

- Two teaspoons of cinnamon, ground.

- One tablespoon of sea salt.

- Half a teaspoon of allspice mix.

- Half a teaspoon of pepper.

- Half a teaspoon of cloves, ground.

- Three pounds of beef, trimmed.

- Two tablespoons of olive oil.

- One medium yellow chopped onion.

- Three sliced cloves of garlic.

- One cup of dry red wine.

- One can of whole tomatoes.

- Five carrots, chopped.

- Two turnips, chopped and peeled.

- Fresh basil to use as garnish.

Instructions to make:

1. Mix together the cinnamon, salt, spice mix, cloves, and pepper into a small mixing bowl, then rub this onto the meat.

2. Heat up the oil in a big pan using a medium heat setting, then add the meat and allow it to cook until it turns slightly brown (about four minutes for each side). Add this meat to your Crock-pot.

3. Add garlic and onion to your pan, stirring and cooking for a couple of minutes, then add the tomatoes and wine, including the tomato juice. Boil this mixture, making sure you scrape the browned pieces and break your tomatoes up. Add this combination to your Crock-pot with the turnips and carrots.

4. Take the beef out of the Crock-pot and slice it into pieces, then serve it with the vegetables and salt, garnishing it with the basil leaves, if desired.

Recipe #17: Crock-pot Picadillo.

Ingredients you need:

- Two pounds of lean beef or bison.

- One tablespoon of olive oil.

- Four ounces of chicken sausage, cooked and diced.

- One tablespoon of powdered chili.

- Two teaspoons of chopped cumin seeds.

- One teaspoon of oregano (dried).

- Half a teaspoon of cinnamon powder.

- Two tablespoons of tomato paste.

- Two tablespoons of vinegar.

- Half a cup of fresh water.

- Two cups of chopped onion.

- Two cups of chopped Anaheim peppers.

- One cup of corn, cooked.

- Half a cup of pitted, thinly sliced olives.

- Five minced garlic cloves.

- One can of chopped tomatoes.

- Half a teaspoon of salt, or more to taste.

- Pepper to taste.

Instructions to make:

1. Heat up the olive oil in a big pan using medium heat, then add the beef or bison with the sausage and cook it together, using a wooden spatula to break up the meat. This should take about six minutes. You may drain the fat with a colander if needed, then put the meat back in the pan.

2. Add the cinnamon, oregano, cumin, and powdered chili, cooking over a medium heat setting and stirring until the mixture is fragrant. This should require a couple of minutes. The next step is to stir in the vinegar, tomato paste, and water until blended thoroughly.

3. Put this mixture of meat into your Crock-pot, then add the garlic, olives, corn, peppers, and onion. Lastly, put in the tomatoes, including the juice that comes with them.

4. Cover this mixture and allow it to cook for eight hours on low or for four hours on high. Add extra salt and pepper if desired.

Recipe #18: Crock-pot Vegetable and Lamb Stew.

Ingredients you need:

- One and a half pounds of boneless lamb, diced into chunks.

- One teaspoon of salt.

- One tablespoon of olive oil.

- Two large white onions sliced thinly.

- Four minced garlic cloves.

- Half a teaspoon of dried oregano.

- Ground pepper as desired.

- One large potato, diced into thick slices.

- Half a pound of trimmed green beans.

- One medium eggplant, diced.

- One medium sized zucchini, diced.

- Five bay leaves.

- One can of diced up tomatoes.

- Three tablespoons of parsley.

Instructions to make:

1. Season the meat with the salt and pepper as you desire, then heat up the oil using a big skillet and medium heat. Now, add half of your meat to the pan, turning and searing it until it's browned for four minutes. Put the meat into your Crock-pot, then add some more oil to the pan and brown the rest of the meat. Put this in the Crock-pot, as well.

2. Add the rest of the oil to the pan, reducing the heat to a low/medium setting, then add onions to the mix, stirring and cooking until they have softened. Now, add the oregano and garlic and stir, cooking for at least a minute. Add the tomatoes to the mixture, simmering it and mashing them with a fork or potato masher. Take this off of the heat and ladle about half of this juice over to the meat.

3. Arrange the chunks of potato in a bottom layer inside of the Crock-pot, seasoning with salt and pepper as you see fit, then add in the zucchini, eggplant, and green beans, seasoning all layers with some pepper and salt. Next, spread the rest of the onion-tomato blend over the veggies and put the bay leaves over the top.

4. Put the lid on the Crock-pot and cook it on a high setting, making the veggies and meat very tender. This should take about four hours. Throw the bay leaves away and serve this with parsley garnish.

Recipe #19: Orange and Olive Pot Roast.

Ingredients you need:

- One pound of small turnips or potatoes.

- Eight carrots, diced into chunks.

- One large yellow sliced onion.

- One can of drained, stewed tomatoes.

- Juice and zest of one orange.

- Four sliced garlic cloves.

- Three bay leaves.

- Three pounds of trimmed chuck roast.

- One teaspoon of sea salt.

- One teaspoon of pepper, to taste.

- Half a cup of black olives, pitted.

Instructions to make:

1. Blend the turnips or potatoes with the onion, carrots, orange juice and zest, tomatoes, bay leaves, and garlic into your Crock-pot. Place the beef over this, then cover with some salt and pepper. Put the lid on and allow this to cook on low for eight hours or on high for four hours.

2. Move the meat over to the counter to cut. Then take the vegetables out and place them in a medium-sized bowl, using a spoon with slots in it.

3. Take fat from the top of the liquid in the Crock-pot, then add the olives to the mix and some more salt, if desired. Cut the meat up and serve it with the sauce and vegetables.

Recipe #20: Crock-pot Vietnamese Chicken Dish.

Ingredients you need:

- Three cups of chicken broth (low sodium).

- Three shallots sliced very thinly.

- A quarter cup of fish sauce.

- Two tablespoons of brown sugar, lightly packed.

- Four Thai chili peppers, sliced very thinly.

- One teaspoon of red pepper, crushed.

- Two teaspoons of zest of lime.

- Four pounds of chicken breast, with bones and skins.

- Two cups of grated carrots.

- Half a cup of lime juice.

- Half a cup of mint (fresh and sliced).

- Half a cup of basil (fresh).

Instructions to make:

1. Mix together the shallots, broth, brown sugar, fish sauce, chili peppers, and zest of a lime into a Crock-pot, then place the chicken into the broth, with the meat side facing down. Let this cook for three hours on high heat or for six hours on low heat.

2. Take the chicken out and move it over to a cutting board, throw the skin out, then shred the chicken. Put the chicken back into the Crock-pot, then add the basil, mint, lime juice, and carrots.

Chapter 3
Delicious Meals for your Health

Along with the overall food quality you ingest on a regular basis, the amount you eat matters when it comes to being healthy. Bringing in the same amount of food calories as your body burns will help your body weight stay at a healthy level over time. If you eat more than you can burn off, however, you will gain weight. As you accumulate extra weight, you heighten your chances of getting a health issue or even more than one. Included in these risks are cancer, diabetes, respiratory problems, hypertension, and heart disease.

Devising a healthy meal plan that is low in extra calories will not only make you feel much better but will help you live a longer life. Let's look at some recipes that will help you accomplish that without sacrificing any taste or enjoyment.

Recipe #21: Southwest Barley and Three Bean Soup.

Ingredients you need:

- One tablespoon of olive oil.

- One big diced onion.

- One diced stalk of celery.

- One large diced carrot.

- Two cups of fresh water.

- Four cups of chicken or vegetable broth.

- A third of a cup of black beans, dried.

- Half a cup of pearl barley.

- A third of a cup of dried beans (great Northern).

- A third of a cup of kidney beans, dried.

- One tablespoon of powdered chili.

- One teaspoon of cumin, ground.

- Half a teaspoon of fresh or dried oregano.

- Salt and pepper to taste.

Instructions to make:

1. Heat up some oil in the Crock-pot, then add in some carrots, celery, and onion, stirring occasionally until it's softened and cooked. Then add the broth, water, black beans, barley, kidney beans, Northern beans, oregano, cumin, and chili powder.

2. Put the lid on the Crock-pot and allow this to cook as long as necessary until the beans are softened. This should require about eight hours on a low heat and four hours on a higher heat setting.

Recipe #22: A Moroccan Lentil Crock-pot Dish.

Ingredients you need:

- Two cups of diced carrots.

- Two cups of diced onions.

- Four minced garlic cloves.

- Two teaspoons of olive oil.

- One teaspoon of cumin, ground.

- One teaspoon of coriander, ground.

- One teaspoon of turmeric, ground.

- A quarter teaspoon of powdered cinnamon.

- A quarter teaspoon of black pepper.

- Six cups of chicken or vegetable broth.

- Two cups of fresh water.

- Three cups of cauliflower florets.

- Two cups of lentils.

- One can of chopped tomatoes.

- Four cups of spinach.

- Half a cup of cilantro.

- Two tablespoons of lemon juice.

- Two tablespoons of crushed tomato.

Instructions to make:

1. Combine the pepper, cinnamon, turmeric, coriander, cumin, oil, garlic, carrots, and onion into your Crock-pot, then add the water, broth, lentils, cauliflower, tomato paste, and tomatoes. Stir all the ingredients together until they are well mixed.

2. Put the lid on and allow it to cook until the lentils have cooked. This should require about 10 hours on a low setting and five hours on high. In the last half hour, add the spinach to the pot. Before you serve it, mix in the lemon juice and cilantro.

Recipe #23: Red Curry Soup with Lentils.

Ingredients you need:

- One tablespoon of olive oil.

- One large chopped onion.

- Three minced cloves of garlic.

- Two tablespoons of ginger, minced.

- One jalapeno, minced and seeded.

- One tablespoon of powdered curry.

- One teaspoon of ground cinnamon.

- One teaspoon of powdered cumin.

- Two bay leaves.

- One cup and a half of red, rinsed lentils.

- Eight cups of chicken broth.

- Three tablespoons of parsley or cilantro.

- Two tablespoons of lemon juice.

- Two tablespoons of chutney, mango flavored.

- Half a cup of plain yogurt.

- Salt and pepper to taste.

Instructions to make:

1. Add some oil, onion, ginger, garlic, curry powder, jalapeno, cumin, bay leaves, and cinnamon to the Crock-pot, stirring it very often.

2. Add the broth and lentils in and put the lid on, allowing the lentils to cook in the juice. Get rid of the bay leaves, then stir in the parsley or cilantro, with the lemon juice. This may be seasoned with pepper, then ladled into bowls and served with chutney and yogurt.

Recipe #24: Traditional Pot Roast Dish.

Ingredients you need:

- One teaspoon of oregano, dried.

- Half a teaspoon of onion flavored salt.

- Half a teaspoon of caraway seeds.

- Half a teaspoon of ground black pepper.

- A quarter teaspoon of garlic salt.

- Four pounds of boneless pork, trimmed.

- Six carrots, peeled and chopped.

- Three potatoes, peeled and chopped.

- Three small quartered onions.

- One and a half cups of broth (beef).

- A third of a cup of flour.

- A third of a cup of fresh water.

- A quarter teaspoon of gravy or browning sauce.

Instructions to make:

1. Mix together the oregano, caraway seeds, onion salt, pepper, and garlic salt, then rub this on the meat. Put plastic wrap over the meat and leave it in the fridge for one night.

2. Put the potatoes, onion, and carrots into your Crock-pot, then add the broth. Take the plastic wrap off the roast and put the roast into the Crock-pot. Put the lid on and cook it until the veggies and meat are nice and tender. This should require between eight and 10 hours.

3. Transfer the vegetables and roast to a platter for serving, tenting it with some tin foil. Pour the leftover cooking juice into a saucepan, mixing water and flour until the sauce is smooth. Stir this into a pan and allow it to boil, stirring and cooking until it has thickened. If you desire to, this is when you should add the gravy or browning sauce. The dish should be served with vegetables and gravy.

Recipe #25: Fantastic Crock-pot Fajitas.

Ingredients you need:

- One and a half pounds of strips of sirloin steak.

- Two tablespoons of olive oil.

- Two tablespoons of lemon juice.

- One minced garlic clove.

- Between one and two teaspoons of cumin.

- Salt and pepper to your preference.

- Half a teaspoon of powdered chili.

- Half a teaspoon of crushed pepper flakes.

- One big white chopped onion.

- One chopped green pepper.

- Eight corn or flour tortillas.

- Tomatoes or lettuce, if desired.

- Salsa, sour cream, shredded cheese for garnish.

Instructions to make:

1. In one large cooking pan, brown the sirloin steak using a medium heat setting, then put the meat and oils into your Crock-pot. Add the garlic, lemon juice, pepper flakes, chili powder, salt, pepper, and cumin.

2. Put the lid on and allow this to cook on a high heat or until the steak is nearly tender. After about three hours, add the onion and green pepper, cooking until the vegetables and meat are fully tender (another hour or so).

3. Next, you should warm up the tortillas, then spoon the vegetables and meat into the tortillas. These can be topped with tomatoes, lettuce, sour cream, salsa, and cheese as desired.

Recipe #26: Pork Roast Teriyaki.

Ingredients you need:

- Three-quarters cup of apple juice, unsweetened.

- Two tablespoons of unrefined sugar.

- Two tablespoons of soy sauce (reduced sodium).

- One teaspoon of powdered ginger.

- One tablespoon of vinegar (white).

- A quarter teaspoon of powdered garlic.

- Salt and pepper to taste.

- Three pounds of boneless pork.

- Two teaspoons of cornstarch.

- Three tablespoons of fresh water.

Instructions to make:

1. Grease up your Crock-pot, then mix together the apple juice, sugar, soy sauce, ginger, vinegar, garlic, salt, and pepper inside. Add the meat and make sure you turn it over to coat it thoroughly. Put the lid on and cook this for about eight hours on low, or until the pork is nice and tender.

2. Take the meat out and put it onto a serving plate, keeping it hot. From the top of the cooking juices, skin the fat and move it over to a saucepan, then bring that to a simmer. Mix the water and cornstarch until the texture is smooth. Stir this gradually into the pot, then boil and allow to thicken. This should be served with the meat.

Recipe #27: Delicious Slow Cooked Winter Stew.

Ingredients you need:

- Two medium chopped and peeled potatoes.

- One pound of stew meat (beef).

- One can of beef broth.

- One can of V8 juice.

- Two stalks of chopped celery.

- Two chopped carrots.

- One medium yellow chopped onion.

- Three bay leaves.

- Half a teaspoon of thyme, dried.

- Half a teaspoon of sea salt, to taste.

- Half a teaspoon of powdered chili.

- A quarter teaspoon of black pepper.

- Two tablespoons of cornstarch.

- One tablespoon of fresh water.

- Half a cup of frozen, thawed peas.

- Half a cup of frozen, thawed corn.

Instructions to make:

- In your Crock-pot, mix together the potatoes, beef, broth, V8, celery, carrots, onion, bay leaves, thyme, salt, chili, and pepper. Put the lid on and allow this to cook for about eight hours on a low setting, or until the meat is soft. Throw the bay leaves away.

- Take a medium sized bowl on the size and mix together the water and cornstarch, stirring until smooth, then add this to the stew. Mix in the peas and corn, then put the lid on. Allow this to cook on a high heat for a half hour, or until it thickens up.

Recipe #28: Onion and Apple Pot Roast.

Ingredients you need:

- Three pounds of beef sirloin, halved.

- One cup of fresh water.

- One teaspoon of flavored salt.

- Half a teaspoon of soy sauce.

- Half a teaspoon of Worcestershire.

- A quarter teaspoon of powdered garlic.

- One large sour apple cut into quarters.

- One big sliced onion.

- Two tablespoons of fresh water.

- Two tablespoons of cornstarch.

- An eighth of a teaspoon of gravy or browning sauce.

Instructions to make:

1. In a large pan that has been oiled, brown the meat on every side. Put this meat into your Crock-pot, then add water to your cooking pan. Stir the water around to loosen up any browned pieces in the pan, then pour this water over the meat. Add soy sauce, garlic powder, Worcestershire sauce, and soy sauce. Add the onion and apple.

2. Put the lid on the Crock-pot and allow it to cook for six hours, letting the meat get nice and tender. Take the meat and onion out of the Crock-pot and let it sit for a while before cutting. Strain the liquid from the Crock-pot into a cooking pan, throwing the apple away.

3. Boil this liquid, cooking it down until it's only two cups, which should take roughly 15 minutes of boiling. Blend the cold water and cornstarch until it's a smooth consistency, then mix in the browning sauce. Stir this into your cooking liquid, boiling it and thickening it up. Serve this with onion and beef.

Recipe #29: Crock-pot Stuffed Peppers.

Ingredients you need:

- Four red peppers, medium sized and sweet.

- One can of rinsed and drained black beans.

- One cup of shredded cheese.

- One cup of chunky salsa.

- One medium yellow onion, diced.

- Half a cup of thawed frozen corn.

- A third of a cup of uncooked brown rice.

- One teaspoon of powdered chili.

- Half a teaspoon of cumin.

- Low-fat sour cream, if desired.

Instructions to make:

1. Cut the tops from the red peppers, throwing away the seeds. In one medium sized mixing bowl, combine the cheese, beans, onion, salsa, rice, corn, cumin, chili powder, and then spoon this blend into the hollowed out peppers.

2. Place these into your Crock-pot, which should have a layer of olive oil to prevent sticking. Cook these for four hours, allowing the peppers to get tender. Check that the filling is hot before taking them out, then serve it with the low-fat sour cream.

Recipe #30: Pumpkin and Black Bean Chili.

Ingredients you need:

- One medium yellow onion, chopped.

- Two tablespoons of virgin olive oil.

- One chopped yellow pepper.

- Three minced garlic cloves.

- Two cans of rinsed and drained black beans.

- One can of pumpkin.

- One can of chopped tomatoes.

- Three cups of chicken broth.

- Two and a half cups of cooked and diced turkey.

- Two teaspoons of parsley, dried and chopped.

- Two teaspoons of powdered chili.

- One and a half teaspoons of cumin.

- One and a half teaspoons of oregano.

- Salt and pepper to taste.

- Chopped avocado and green onion, if desired.

Instructions to make:

1. In one big pan, heat up the oil at a medium setting, then add the pepper and onion. Stir and cook these ingredients until tender, then add the garlic and cook for another minute.

2. Move this over to the Crock-pot, then blend in the rest of the ingredients. Allow this to cook with the lid on for about five hours. When it's done, top it with green onion and avocado, if desired.

Chapter 4
Unique Crock-pot Dishes to Try at Home

Weight gain is just one of the symptoms of bad nutrition. Not getting enough nutrients, or getting too much of certain ones, can also cause serious issues with your health. For example, not getting enough calcium can increase your risk of developing osteoporosis or other bone problems, and too many bad fats can increase your risk of cardiovascular diseases. In addition, not getting enough vegetables and fruit in your diet is shown to increase your risk of developing cancer. Eating enough food from a large variety of food sources will help your body get the nutrition it requires to stay healthy. Here are some more recipes to get you started!

Recipe #31: Italian Peppers and Chicken.

Ingredients you need:

- One jar of spaghetti sauce, garden style.

- One medium, sliced onion.

- A quarter cup of Parmesan cheese, grated.

- Two minced garlic cloves.

- One teaspoon of basil, dried.

- One teaspoon of oregano, dried.

- Salt and pepper, to taste.

- Half a cup of red peppers.

- Half a cup of sweet yellow peppers.

- Half a cup of small green peppers.

- Six skinless, boneless chicken breasts.

- Cooked black bean pasta.

Instructions to make:

1. Blend together the spaghetti sauce, onion, parmesan cheese, garlic, basil, oregano, salt, and pepper together, then add the peppers to the Crock-pot. Put the chicken into the Crock-pot and smother it with the sauce mix.

2. Put the lid on the Crock-pot and allow it to cook on low for four hours, or until a thermometer says 165 degrees F. This can be served with the black bean pasta or another healthier pasta substitute.

Recipe #32: Pineapple Mango Chicken Wraps.

Ingredients you need:

- Two mangoes, chopped and peeled.

- One and a half cups of canned or fresh pineapple pieces.

- Two large chopped tomatoes.

- One red onion, diced finely.

- Two seeded, chopped Anaheim peppers.

- Two finely chopped green onions.

- One tablespoon of lime juice.

- One tablespoon of raw sugar.

- Four pounds of chicken breasts with bones.

- Three teaspoons of sea salt.

- A quarter cup of brown sugar.

- Tortilla shells.

- Some fresh cilantro, if desired.

Instructions to make:

1. Mix together the mangoes, pineapple, tomatoes, onion, peppers, green onion, lime juice, and sugar into a large mixing bowl. Then put the chicken into your Crock-pot, topping it

with sugar and salt. Add the mango mix to this, then allow it to cook for six hours on low heat, or until the meat has softened.

2. Take the chicken out of the pot and allow it to cool down slightly. Strain the juices from the cooking, keeping half a cup of the juice with the mango mixture. Get rid of the extra juices. Once this has cooled down enough, de-bone the chicken, throwing the bones away. Shred the chicken, then return the mango mixture and chicken, along with the juices to the Crock-pot. Serve this in tortillas.

Recipe #33: Super Green and Healthy Soup.

Ingredients you need:

- Two tablespoons of olive oil, or more to taste.

- Two large chopped onions.

- Salt and pepper, to taste.

- Two tablespoons of fresh water.

- Four cups of fresh water (kept separate).

- One cup of brown or green lentils.

- Eight chard leaves, large.

- One yellow potato, cleaned.

- 12 cups of spinach, de-stemmed.

- Four scallions, diced.

- Five cups of vegetable broth.

- Two cups of broccoli, chopped.

- One tablespoon of cumin.

- Half a teaspoon of coriander.

- Black pepper to taste.

- Two tablespoons of mint, fresh.

- One cup of cilantro.

- Half a minced jalapeno pepper.

- One tablespoon of lemon juice.

- Feta cheese, crumbled.

Instructions to make:

1. Warm up two tablespoons of olive oil in a big pan using a high heat setting, then add the onions and salt, stirring often. Wait for the onions to brown, then lower the heat and add some water, then cover the pan. Cook this, stirring often until the skillet cools.

2. At the same time, clean your lentils, mixing them with four cups of fresh water in a pot. Allow this to boil, then reduce that heat until it's simmering. Then cover this and allow it to cook for 15 to 20 minutes.

3. Cut the white ribs off of your chard, then chop them and cut the ribs (kept separately). Dice the potato into half inch cubes, and chop the spinach finely. Set all of this aside for now. As soon as the lentils have been cooking for 20 minutes, add the broth, scallions, potato, salt, and chard ribs, then simmer it again. Put the lid on and allow this to cook for 10 to 15 minutes or so.

4. Stir the leaves of chard, coriander, cumin, and broccoli into the mix. As soon as your onions have been caramelized, mix some liquid with them, then add this all to the pot. Return

this to a simmer, and allow it to cook with the lid on for another five minutes.

5. Add the pepper, jalapeno, mint, cilantro, and spinach, then return this to a light simmer with the lid on again. Allow it to cook for about five minutes or until the spinach is slightly tender. Add a tablespoon of lemon juice, and add more if you wish to. Serve with feta cheese.

Recipe #34: Zesty Beef and Orange Dish.

Ingredients you need:

- One pound of sirloin steak, cut into strips.

- Two cups of shiitake mushrooms, fresh.

- One diced onion.

- Three hot chilies, dried.

- A quarter cup of brown sugar.

- A quarter cup of fresh orange juice.

- A quarter cup of soy sauce, reduced sodium.

- One tablespoon of cornstarch.

- Three tablespoons of apple cider vinegar.

- One tablespoon of ginger, minced.

- One tablespoon of sesame oil.

- Four minced garlic cloves.

- One cup of snow peas, fresh.

- One tablespoon of orange rind.

- Cooked brown rice.

Instructions to make:

1. Put the meat into the Crock-pot, then add in the chilies, onion, and mushroom. In a medium sized bowl on the size, mix together the garlic, oil, ginger, cornstarch, vinegar, soy sauce, orange juice and brown sugar, then pour this over the beef.

2. Put the lid on the Crock-pot and let it cook for six hours, then add the peas when the meal is almost ready. Stir the orange peel in and then serve this with the hot brown rice.

Recipe #35: Couscous and Chicken dish.

Ingredients you need:

- Two sweet potatoes, peeled and chopped.

- One red pepper, chopped coarsely.

- One and a half pounds of skinless, boneless chicken.

- One can of undrained, stewed tomatoes.

- Half a cup of mango or peach salsa.

- A quarter cup of raisins.

- Salt and pepper to taste.

- A quarter teaspoon of cumin.

- A quarter teaspoon of cinnamon.

- A quarter teaspoon of pepper.

- One cup of couscous, uncooked.

- One cup of fresh water (for the couscous).

Instructions to make:

1. In your Crock-pot, add the red peppers, sweet potatoes, and chicken. Mix together the seasonings, raisins, salsa, and tomatoes in a medium mixing bowl. Pour this blend over the meat, then cook with a lid on for four hours, until the chicken and potatoes are tender.

2. When the meal is 10 minutes from being ready, cook the couscous by boiling the water then stirring in the couscous. Take it off the heat and allow it to stand with a lid on for five minutes.

3. Take the chicken out of the Crock-pot and shred it coarsely using two forks, then put the chicken back into the Crock-pot. Stir this together to mix and serve with the couscous.

Recipe #36: Crock-pot French Onion Soup.

Ingredients you need:

- Two tablespoons of cold butter, chopped.

- Two tablespoons of olive oil, extra virgin.

- Eight fresh thyme sprigs.

- Four smashed garlic cloves.

- Two sliced pounds of yellow onion.

- Two sliced pounds of red onion.

- Salt and pepper to taste.

- One bay leaf.

- Four cups of beef or vegetable broth.

- A quarter cup of dry sherry.

- Eight slices of baguette bread, toasted.

- One cup of shredded Swiss cheese.

Instructions to make:

1. To prepare the French onion soup, spread butter in your Crock-pot, then add the bay leaf, garlic, thyme, oil, and onions last. Cover with salt and pepper as desired, then put the lid on and let it cook for eight hours on high.

2. Boil the sherry and broth in a separate pan, the, remove the thyme and bay leaf from your Crock-pot. Pour the broth in and allow it to cook without a lid for about 10 minutes or so.

3. Broil the baguette slices with the cheese on top so that it melts, then divide the soup into bowls and top with the toast and cheese.

Recipe #37: Crock-pot Berry and Turkey Compote.

Ingredients you need:

- Salt and pepper to taste.

- Half a teaspoon of powdered garlic.

- Half a teaspoon of thyme, dried.

- Four pounds of boneless turkey meat.

- A third of a cup of fresh water.

- Two medium, chopped apples, peeled.

- Two cups of raspberries, fresh.

- Two cups of blueberries, fresh.

- One cup of grape juice, white.

- A quarter teaspoon of pepper flakes.

- A quarter teaspoon of powdered ginger.

Instructions to make:

1. Blend together the pepper, thyme, garlic powder, and salt, then smother it over the turkey meat. Put this into your Crock-pot, pouring water around it. Allow it to cook for four hours on low or until the turkey reads 165 degrees on a meat thermometer.

2. Take the turkey out of the Crock-pot, then create a tinfoil tent around it. Allow this to sit for 10 minutes, then slice. While it's sitting, mix together the fruit and grape juice, making a sauce to serve with the turkey.

Recipe #38: Crock-pot Pork Stew.

Ingredients you need:

- One pound of pork tenderloins, chopped.

- Salt and pepper to taste.

- Two sliced carrots, large.

- Two ribs of coarsely chopped celery.

- One medium, chopped onion.

- Three cups of broth.

- Two tablespoons of crushed tomato.

- A third a cup of pitted plums, dried and chopped.

- Four minced garlic cloves.

- Two bay leaves.

- One sprig of thyme, fresh.

- One sprig of rosemary, fresh.

- A third a cup of olives, optional.

- Parsley to garnish, if desired.

- Mashed potatoes, if desired.

Instructions to make:

1. Sprinkle the meat with however much salt and pepper you wish, then move it to the Crock-pot. Add the onion, celery, and carrots. Whisk together the tomato paste and broth in a mixing bowl, then cover the vegetables with it.

2. Add the thyme, rosemary, bay leaves, garlic, and plums, then add the olives last. Allow this to cook for six hours or until the veggies and meat are tender. Throw out the thyme, rosemary, and bay leaves and serve with parsley and potatoes.

Recipe #39: Crock-pot Seafood Dish.

Ingredients you need:

- One can of undrained, diced tomatoes.

- Two chopped onions, medium.

- Three chopped celery stalks.

- One can of clam juice.

- One can of crushed tomato.

- Half a cup of broth or white wine.

- Five minced garlic cloves.

- One tablespoon of vinegar, red wine.

- One tablespoon of virgin olive oil.

- Two teaspoons of oregano or Italian seasoning.

- One or two bay leaves.

- Half a teaspoon of raw sugar.

- One pound of haddock fish, chopped.

- One pound of raw shrimp, peeled.

- One can of chopped clams.

- One can of crab meat.

- Two tablespoons of parsley, minced.

Instructions to make:

1. To make this dish, just mix the diced tomatoes, onions, celery, clam juice, crushed tomato, broth or wine, garlic, vinegar, olive, Italian, bay leaves, and sugar. Allow this to simmer with a lid on for five hours.

2. Add the seafood to the pot, then cook with the lid on for another half hour, or once the shrimp and fish look cooked. Take out the bay leaf and serve with fresh parsley.

Recipe #40: Ham and Black-Eyed Peas.

Ingredients you need:

- One can of dried black-eyed peas.

- Half a pound of ham, boneless, cooked and chopped.

- One finely chopped medium onion.

- One red pepper, also finely chopped.

- Five cooked bacon strips, crumbled.

- One large chopped jalapeno pepper.

- Two minced garlic cloves.

- Half a teaspoon of powdered cumin.

- One teaspoon of chicken bouillon cubes.

- Half a teaspoon of cayenne pepper.

- Salt and pepper to taste.

- Six cups of water.

- Fresh, minced cilantro, if desired.

- Brown cooked rice, hot.

Instructions to make:

1. Soak the black-eyed peas as instructed on the package, then move them over to the Crock-pot. Add the rest of the ingredients on the list and allow it to cook for seven hours. This can be served with rice and cilantro.

Chapter 5
More Recipes to Enjoy

If eating a healthy diet is new to you, it's best to do it gradually, then your habits can change over time instead of all at once, helping you get healthier as you go along. For instance, you can swap out soda for lemon water, and cut out adding extra sugar to your food. Choosing lean meats, rather than the fatty cuts, and going for whole grains rather than the refined options, can help you get more fiber and cut out extra fat. Fresh vegetables and fruits are always better than canned, and eating cucumber slices with hummus instead of chips and dip is also a great change. Here are some more recipes to help you get healthy and fit!

Recipe #41: Veggie and Beef Dish.

Ingredients you need:

- One and a half pounds of boneless cubed beef.

- Three potatoes, peeled and chopped.

- Three cups of fresh water.

- One and a half cups of baby carrots.

- One can of undiluted tomato soup.

- One chopped onion.

- One chopped celery stalk.

- Two tablespoons of Worcestershire.

- One tablespoon of gravy or browning sauce.

- Two teaspoons of beef bouillon.

- One minced garlic clove.

- One teaspoon of raw sugar.

- Salt and pepper, to taste.

- A quarter cup of cornstarch.

- Three-quarters of a cup of fresh water.

- Two cups of thawed frozen peas.

Instructions to make:

1. Place the celery, onion, soup, carrots, water, potatoes, beef, Worcestershire sauce, gravy if desired, bouillon cubes, sugar, garlic, salt, and pepper in your Crock-pot. Cover and allow this to cook until the beef is nice and tender, for about eight hours.

2. Mix together the water and cornstarch, blending in a bowl until the mixture is smooth. Stir this into the Crock-pot gradually, then add the peas. Put the lid on and let this cook until thick. This should require about a half hour.

Recipe #42: Crock-pot Sunday Chicken Meal.

Ingredients you need:

- Two chopped carrots, small.

- Half an onion, chopped.

- Half a celery stalk, chopped.

- One cup of fresh green beans.

- Two halved small potatoes.

- Two chicken breasts with the bones still in.

- Two strips of cooked bacon, crumbled.

- One cup of warm water.

- One teaspoon of chicken flavored bouillon.

- Salt and pepper to taste.

- A quarter teaspoon of basil, dried.

- A quarter teaspoon of thyme, dried.

Instructions to make:

1. Blend the carrots, onion, celery, green beans, potatoes, chicken, and bacon into your Crock-pot, then add the salt and pepper, water, bouillon, and herbs but don't stir. Put the lid on and allow this to cook for eight hours on low, or until the meat and vegetables are tender. Take the vegetables and chicken out, then thicken up the remaining juices to create a gravy.

Recipe #43: Crock-pot Beef Tips.

Ingredients you need:

- One pound of mushrooms, sliced up.

- One small sliced onion.

- One beef steak, cubed (one pound).

- Salt and pepper to taste.

- Two teaspoons of olive oil.

- A third a cup of beef broth or dry red wine.

- Two cups of beef broth.

- One tablespoon of Worcestershire.

- Two tablespoons of cornstarch.

- A fourth a cup of fresh water.

- Mashed potatoes to serve with, if desired.

Instructions to make:

1. Place the onions and mushroom into a Crock-pot, then season the meat with as much salt and pepper as desired. In one large pan, heat up the olive oil, browning the meat in pieces, then adding more oil if you need to. Move the meat over to the Crock-pot.

2. Add the dry red wine to the pan, stirring to get the brown bits off the bottom, then add the Worcestershire sauce and broth to pour over the meat. Allow this to cook with the lid on for eight hours.

3. Mix together the cold water and cornstarch in a medium mixing bowl, then gradually stir this into the Crock-pot. Cover and cook for a half hour, or until the gravy has gotten thicker. This can be served with hot mashed potatoes.

Recipe #44: Crock-pot Coconut Chicken.

This is an Asian-inspired dish that can be made spicy if you desire. To make it spicy, just add cayenne pepper or crushed pepper flakes and serve with Sriracha sauce.

Ingredients you need:

- Half a cup of coconut milk, light.

- Two tablespoons of raw brown sugar.

- Two tablespoons of soy sauce.

- Two minced garlic cloves.

- A teaspoon of powdered cloves.

- Six boneless chicken breasts or thighs.

- Six tablespoons of coconut shreds, toasted.

Instructions to make:

1. Combine the coconut milk, brown sugar, soy sauce, garlic, and cloves in a bowl, blending together. Then put the chicken into the Crock-pot, pouring the coconut milk sauce over it. Put the lid on and let this cook for five hours, then serve with coconut shreds.

Recipe #45: BBQ Sauce Chicken.

Ingredients you need:

- Six chicken thighs, boneless and skinless.

- Half a teaspoon of chicken seasoning.

- One large onion, finely chopped.

- One can of undrained, chopped tomatoes.

- One can of tomato sauce.

- Half a cup of barbecue sauce.

- A quarter cup of unsweetened orange juice.

- One teaspoon of powdered garlic.

- One teaspoon of oregano, dried.

- Half a teaspoon of hot sauce, if desired.

- Half a teaspoon of pepper, or more.

- Brown rice on the side, cooked.

Instructions to make:

1. Place the chicken into the Crock-pot, then cover it with the chicken seasoning. Add the tomatoes and onion on top. Mix together the orange juice, seasonings, tomato sauce, and then pour it over the meat.

2. Allow this to cook with a lid on for six hours, or until the meat is done. You can serve this with rice, if desired.

Recipe #46: Chili Sauce Meat Loaf.

Ingredients you need:

- One large, finely chopped onion.

- Half a cup of bread crumbs, seasoned.

- One small chopped pepper, green.

- Two large eggs, beaten slightly.

- Half a cup of chili sauce.

- Two tablespoons of mustard, spicy brown.

- Four minced garlic cloves.

- Salt and pepper, to taste.

- A quarter teaspoon of oregano, dried.

- A quarter teaspoon of basil, dried.

- Two pounds of 90 percent lean beef.

- Extra chili sauce, if desired.

Instructions to make:

1. Cut out four thin, long sheets of heavy duty tin foil, then cross them so they look like wheel spokes. Add the strips to the bottom and sides of your Crock-pot, coating them with cooking spray.

2. Combine the onion, bread crumbs, pepper, eggs, chili sauce, mustard, garlic, oregano, basil, and salt and pepper in a big mixing bowl. Add the meat to this, mixing lightly but being very thorough. Shape this into a round loaf that measures about 9 inches. Put this loaf in the middle of the strips inside of your Crock-pot.

3. Cook this with the lid on for four hours, adding some extra chili sauce over the meat if desired. Allow it to stand for about 10 minutes before taking it out. Use the foil to remove the meatloaf and put it onto a serving platter.

4. This dish can be frozen in a greased, shallow glass dish. In order to use again, allow these to thaw partially in the fridge overnight, then take it out a half hour before you want to bake it.

Recipe #47: Rice and Beef Cabbage Rolls.

Ingredients you need:

- 12 full leaves of cabbage.

- One cup of brown rice, cooked.

- A quarter cup of onion, finely chopped.

- One large egg, beaten slightly.

- A quarter cup of low-fat milk.

- Salt and pepper to taste.

- One pound of lean meat, beef.

- One can of tomato sauce.

- One tablespoon of lemon juice.

- One tablespoon of raw brown sugar.

- One teaspoon of Worcestershire.

Instructions to make:

1. To make this recipe, cook the cabbage in batches in boiling water. This should require about five minutes and will be done when the leaves are crisp-tender. Drain these and allow them to cool slightly. Cut the vein off the cabbage leaves, resulting in a V-shape.

2. Combine the onion, rice, egg, salt, pepper, and milk in a large mixing bowl, then add the meat. Mix this a bit but make sure you do it thoroughly. Add a quarter cup of this meat mixture onto each leaf of cabbage. Pull these together, then cut the leaf edges so that they overlap. Fold it over the filling, fold in the sides, and roll it all up.

3. Put six of these rolls into the Crock-pot with the seam facing down. In a separate bowl, mix together the ingredients for the sauce (the tomato sauce, lemon juice, sugar, and Worcestershire sauce). Pour half of this over the rolls of cabbage in the Crock-pot. Add the rest of the rolls and the rest of the sauce, then cook it for eight hours.

Recipe #48: Spicy Carne Dish.

This is one for the spicy meat lovers in your family. When you cook this, you're sure to have leftovers for your loved ones to enjoy again. Here's how you make this exciting meal.

Ingredients you need:

- One bottle of beer.

- A quarter cup of flour.

- Two tablespoons of crushed tomato paste.

- One full jalapeno pepper, chopped and seeded.

- Four teaspoons of Worcestershire.

- One bay leaf.

- Three teaspoons of pepper flakes.

- Two teaspoons of powdered chili.

- One teaspoon of powdered cumin.

- Salt and pepper to taste.

- Half a teaspoon of paprika.

- Two minced garlic cloves.

- Half a teaspoon of vinegar, red wine.

- Liquid smoke, if desired.

- One pork shoulder, boneless, chopped.

- Two large chopped potatoes.

- One chopped onion.

- Brown rice or tortillas.

- Lime wedges and cilantro, if desired.

Instructions to make:

1. In a Crock-pot, blend together the beer, flour, tomato paste, jalapeno, Worcestershire, bay leaf, pepper flakes, chili, cumin, salt, and pepper, paprika, and garlic. Mix in the potatoes, pork, and onion.

2. Put the lid on and let this cook for eight hours, then throw away the bay leaf, take the fat off of the cooking fluids, then shred the meat using two forks. This can be served with rice or tortillas and garnished with lime and cilantro.

Recipe #49: Turkey Breasts and Herbs.

This is a classic favorite. To make it healthier, you can substitute the sugar with honey or simply leave it out altogether. Here's how to make this great dish.

Ingredients you need:

- One can of chicken broth.

- Half a cup of lemon juice.

- A quarter cup of sage, fresh.

- A quarter cup of brown sugar.

- A quarter cup of thyme leaves, fresh.

- A quarter cup of lime juice.

- A quarter cup of apple cider vinegar.

- A quarter cup of olive oil.

- One packet of onion soup powder.

- Two tablespoons of mustard, Dijon.

- One tablespoon of marjoram, fresh.

- Two teaspoons of paprika.

- One teaspoon of powdered garlic.

- Salt and pepper to taste.

- Two boneless turkey breasts.

Instructions to make:

1. Blend the chicken broth, lemon juice, sage, brown sugar, thyme, lime juice, vinegar, olive, onion soup powder, mustard, marjoram, paprika, powdered garlic, and salt and pepper in a blender. Pour this sauce into a plastic bag with a Ziplock, then add the meat. Seal this bag and shake to coat the turkey, then leave it in the fridge overnight.

2. Move the turkey and allow it to marinade in the Crock-pot, then cook on high for four hours.

Recipe #50: Caribbean Style Pot Roast.

This dish is just exotic enough to excite your guests but familiar enough to be an instant favorite. Whip this out for an ordinary family dinner, or to bring to a potluck. Here's how to make it:

Ingredients you need:

- Two sweet potatoes, chopped into cubes.

- Two large sliced carrots.

- A quarter cup of chopped celery.

- One beef roast, boneless (about 2 pounds).

- One tablespoon of olive oil.

- One large chopped onion.

- Two minced garlic cloves.

- One tablespoon of flour.

- One tablespoon of brown sugar.

- One tablespoon of regular sugar.

- One teaspoon of powdered cumin.

- Salt and pepper, to taste.

- One teaspoon of coriander, ground.

- One teaspoon of chili powder.

- One teaspoon of oregano, dried.

- Half a teaspoon of cinnamon.

- One teaspoon of orange rind.

- One teaspoon of baking cocoa.

- One can of tomato juice or sauce.

Instructions to make:

1. Put the celery, carrots, and potatoes into the Crock-pot. In one large pan, brown the meat on every side, then move it over to the Crock-pot.

2. Using the same pan, cook the onion in the meat drippings until it gets soft. Add the garlic cloves and cook for another minute or so. Blend together the sugar, flour, seasoning, cocoa, and orange rind, then add some tomato sauce. Add this all to the pan and allow it to heat. Pour this sauce over the meat. Cover this with a lid and let it cook for eight hours in the Crock-pot.

Chapter 6
Healthy Crock-pot Food Anyone can Make

As mentioned before, eating plenty of fruits and vegetables will give you plentiful health benefits. Those who make sure to eat more fruit and vegetables as part of a balanced diet have a lowered risk of issues such as obesity and other chronic illnesses. Let's look at some great recipes to keep you healthy and thriving, while staying in great shape!

Recipe #51: Classic Crock-pot Pepper Steak.

This is a familiar dish that most have tried, but with a unique spin on it. This can be left in your Crock-pot to simmer all day while you're away at work.

Ingredients you need:

- Three bounds of round top beef roast.

- One large sliced onion, cut in half.

- One large pepper, green and chopped.

- One large red pepper, chopped.

- One cup of fresh water.

- Four cloves of minced garlic.

- A third of a cup of cornstarch.

- Half a cup of soy sauce.

- Two teaspoons of raw sugar.

- Two teaspoons of powdered ginger.

- Eight cups of brown rice, cooked and warm.

Instructions to make:

1. Put the meat, peppers, and onion into your Crock-pot, then add the fresh water and minced garlic. Allow this to cook with a lid on for about eight hours, or until the roast feels tender with your fork.

2. Take the beef out and place it on a cutting board, then move the cooking juices and vegetables over to a large pan. Boil this, then mix together the soy sauce, cornstarch, ginger, and sugar until they blend smoothly. Add this to the mixture of vegetables. Boil this again while constantly stirring it, then cook it for another two minutes, stirring the whole time, until it thickens up.

3. Slice the beef up and stir the meat into the sauce, making sure it's fully heated through before serving with hot rice.

Recipe #52: Crock-pot Lemon Chicken Dish.

Lemon chicken is something most of us have tried, but it usually requires a lot more work than this tasty, easy Crock-pot recipe. Here's how you make it.

Ingredients you need:

- Six halves of chicken breasts, with the bones still in.

- One teaspoon of oregano, dried.

- Half a teaspoon of seasoning salt.

- Half a teaspoon of pepper.

- Two tablespoons of butter.

- A quarter cup of fresh water.

- Three tablespoons of fresh lemon juice.

- Two minced garlic cloves.

- One teaspoon of granulated chicken bouillon.

- Two teaspoons of parsley, minced and fresh.

- Brown rice, cooked and hot.

Instructions to make:

1. To make this dish, first, make sure the chicken is patted dry with paper. Mix together the salt, pepper, oregano, and rub it over the meat. In a pan, using medium heat, cook the chicken

using butter until it's brown, then move this over to the Crock-pot.

2. Add the fresh water, garlic, lemon juice, and bouillon granules to the pan, then boil it. Make sure you stir to loosen up the brown pieces on the bottom. Pour this over the meat.

3. Put the lid on the Crock-pot and allow it to cook for about six hours. Baste the chicken using the juices from the cooking, then add some fresh parsley if desired. Put the lid on and cook this for another half hour, or until the juices in the meat are clear. Serve this with brown rice. You may thicken the cooking juices to make a gravy, if desired.

Recipe #53: Barbecue Spaghetti Dish.

Barbecue is not something you'd typically think of as connected to spaghetti, but it goes together fantastically. Here's how you make this wonderful Southern-style dish.

Ingredients you need:

- One pound of turkey, lean and ground.

- Two chopped onions.

- One cup of mushrooms, sliced.

- One chopped green pepper.

- Two cloves of minced garlic.

- One can of undrained, diced tomatoes.

- One can of crushed tomatoes or tomato paste.

- One cup of low sodium ketchup.

- Half a cup of beef broth.

- Two tablespoons of Worcestershire.

- Two tablespoons of raw brown sugar.

- One tablespoon of powdered cumin.

- Two teaspoons of powdered chili.

- Hot, fresh spaghetti, cooked.

Instructions to make:

1. To cook this, prepare the onions, turkey, green peppers, and mushrooms over medium heat. Brown the meat, then add the garlic for the last minute of cooking. Drain the meat.

2. Move the ground meat over to your Crock-pot, then stir in the tomato paste, tomatoes, tomato sauce, broth, Worcestershire, ketchup, cumin, chili powder, and brown sugar. Put the lid on and let this cook for about five hours, or until the vegetables are soft. Serve this dish with the hot pasta.

Recipe #54: Flavorful Chicken and Rice Dish.

Ingredients you need:

- One can of cream of chicken soup, undiluted.

- Three tablespoons of flour.

- A quarter teaspoon of black pepper.

- Cayenne pepper, if desired.

- One pound of chicken breasts, boneless and diced.

- One stalk of celery, chopped.

- Half a cup of green pepper, diced.

- A quarter cup of onion, chopped.

- One package of thawed frozen peas.

- Two tablespoons of drained, diced pimientos.

- Brown rice, cooked and hot.

Instructions to make:

1. In your Crock-pot, blend together the flour, soup, cayenne, and black pepper until the mixture is nice and smooth, then add the chicken meat, green pepper, onion, and celery. Put the lid of the Crock-pot on and cook this for eight hours. Stir the pimientos and peas in last, then cook again for another half hour. This should be served with fresh brown rice.

Recipe #55: Chicken Sausage and Lentil Stew.

This dish is healthy and hearty and will warm you in the winter months. This can be served with rolls or cornbread to help you soak up all of the delicious juices.

Ingredients you need:

- One carton of chicken broth, reduced sodium if possible.

- One can of undrained, diced tomatoes.

- Three cooked chicken sausage links, chopped.

- One cup of rinsed dried lentils.

- One chopped medium onion.

- One chopped medium carrot.

- One celery stalk, chopped.

- Two cloves of minced garlic.

- Half a teaspoon of thyme, dried.

Instructions to make:

1. The instructions for this tasty dish are very simple. Just mix together the broth, tomatoes, sausage, lentils, onion, carrot, celery, garlic, and thyme into a Crock-pot. Put the lid on and let it cook for 10 hours while you are at work. You will know it's done when the lentils are soft.

Recipe #56: Shredded, Spicy Crock-pot Chicken.

Mexican food is delicious, but it often comes with a lot of extra calories and fat. This dish, however, is tasty and healthy. You can serve this with tortillas, beans, rice, and chunky salsa on the side. You may also substitute pork or beef for the chicken, according to your family's tastes.

Ingredients you need:

- Two tablespoons of olive oil.

- One pound of chicken thighs, boneless.

- One pound of chicken breasts, boneless.

- Three cups of chicken broth, low sodium.

- Six chopped green onions.

- One chopped medium pepper, green.

- Two tablespoons of powdered cumin.

- One tablespoon of powdered garlic.

- One tablespoon of powdered chili.

- One tablespoon of paprika.

- One teaspoon of cayenne.

- Half a teaspoon of sea salt.

- Half a teaspoon of pepper.

- One chopped plum tomato.

Instructions to make:

1. Using a large pan, heat up the oil, then brown the chicken in sections. Move it over to your Crock-pot, then add a cup of broth to the same pan. Cook the broth, making sure to loosen the browned pieces from the pan's bottom.

2. Add the green pepper and onions, stirring and cooking for about five minutes or until the veggies are soft. Add the seasonings, then cook for another couple minutes. Add the tomatoes and the rest of the broth, then pour this mixture over the meat. Put the lid on and cook for five hours.

3. Take the chicken out of the Crock-pot and let it cool down. Once it has cooled enough, shred it using two forks, then put it into the Crock-pot again. Cook with the lid on for 20 minutes more to heat, and serve using a slotted ladle or spoon. You can freeze this mixture using Tupperware. To serve again, just thaw it in the fridge for one night and heat it up in a saucepan with some broth.

Recipe #57: Italian Style Crock-pot Roast.

This roast is classic but with a twist, the aromatic herbs and spices lend it an exotic, Moroccan vibe and taste. It's a new take on something familiar and great that we all love. Here's how you make it.

Ingredients you need:

- One stick of cinnamon.

- Six peppercorns, whole.

- Three allspice berries, whole.

- Two teaspoons of olive oil.

- One beef roast, boneless.

- Two stalks of celery, chopped.

- Two carrots, chopped.

- One large chopped onion.

- Four minced garlic cloves.

- One cup of beef broth or dry sherry.

- One can of tomatoes, crushed.

- Half a teaspoon of sea salt.

- Egg noodles and parsley on the side, if desired.

Instructions to make:

1. To make this, place the stick of cinnamon, whole peppercorns, allspice, and cloves into a cheesecloth, then gather the corners to enclose them and tie it up with kitchen twine.

2. Using a large pan, heat up the oil, then brown the meat and move it over to the Crock-pot. Add in the spice bag, carrots, and celery. Add your onion to that same pan, stirring and cooking until it's soft. Add the garlic for the last minute, stirring.

3. Add the broth or sherry, bringing it to a strong boil, the stir and cook this until the liquid is only about a cup. Add the salt and tomatoes, then pour this over the veggies and meat.

4. Cook this with a lid on for seven hours. Take the roast out of the Crock-pot and keep it warm, throw away the spice bag and get the fat off the top of the sauce. Serve this with noodles, sauce, and parsley.

Recipe #58: Crock-pot Chicken Cacciatore.

If you have a hectic day planned and don't have time to cook, this dish will be your new best friend. Come home from work and find your house filled with this delicious dinner smell. Here's how to make it.

Ingredients you need:

- Two thinly sliced medium onions.

- One fryer chicken, skin removed and chopped.

- Two cloves of minced garlic.

- Two teaspoons of oregano spice, dried.

- Salt and pepper to taste.

- Half a teaspoon of basil, dried.

- One can of undrained, diced tomatoes.

- One can of tomato sauce.

- One can of mushrooms.

- Half a cup of water or white wine.

- Pasta on the side, cooked and hot.

- One bay leaf.

Instructions to make:

1. Add the onions to your Crock-pot first, then the seasonings, chicken, tomato sauce, tomatoes, wine, and mushrooms. Put the lid on your Crock-pot and allow to cook on a low heat for eight hours. You will know it's done when the chicken is tender. Serve this with the sauce and hot, fresh pasta. You may serve with fresh herbs and cheese, as well.

Recipe #59: Day-Long Crock-pot Brisket and Potatoes.

The Crock-pot was probably invented just to make this dish. It's savory, sweet, and perfect. This is ideal to use with either flat cut or first cut brisket meat due to their low-fat content.

Ingredients you need:

- Two peeled and diced potatoes, medium sized.

- Two sliced stalks of celery.

- Three pounds of beef brisket.

- One tablespoon of olive oil.

- One large sliced onion.

- Two minced garlic cloves.

- One can of beer.

- Half a teaspoon of granulated beef bouillon.

- Three-quarters cup of stewed tomatoes.

- A third of a cup of tomato paste.

- Half a cup of vinegar, red wine.

- Three tablespoons of mustard.

- Three tablespoons of raw brown sugar.

- Three tablespoons of soy sauce with low sodium.

- Two tablespoons of healthy molasses.

- Half a teaspoon of ground paprika.

- One bay leaf.

- Salt and pepper to taste.

Instructions to make:

1. Put the celery and potatoes into your Crock-pot, then cut the meat in half. Using a large pan, brown the meat using oil, then move it over to the Crock-pot. Using the same skillet, cook the onion until it's soft and translucent. Add the garlic and cook for another minute, then add this to the Crock-pot, as well.

2. Add the bouillon granules and beer to the pan, stirring to loosen any browned pieces stuck to the bottom of the pan. Pour this blend over your meat. Mix together the rest of the ingredients in a large mixing bowl, then add them to the Crock-pot.

3. Cover all of this with a lid and let it cook for 10 hours. Slice the meat thinly, throw away the bay leaf, and serve while it's hot.

Recipe #60: Cinnamon and Apple Pork Loin.

This one is reminiscent of a desert or the Christmas season, but you can enjoy it anytime! It's great in the fall or winter and fills your entire home with a great smell. You can serve it with mashed potatoes on the side.

Ingredients you need:

- Three pounds of boneless pork roast.

- Half a teaspoon of salt.

- Half a teaspoon of pepper.

- One tablespoon of olive oil.

- Three apples, sliced, peeled, and chopped.

- A quarter cup of raw honey.

- One red onion, sliced and halved.

- One tablespoon of cinnamon powder.

- Fresh parsley on the side, if desired.

Instructions to make:

1. Sprinkle the meat with as much salt and pepper as you wish. In a big pan, brown the meat using oil, then allow it to slightly cool before proceeding. Using a knife, cut about 16 slots into the meat. These should be about 3 inches deep and you can insert an apple slice into every one of them.

2. Put the remaining apples into your Crock-pot, then place the meat over these. Cover the entire thing with drizzled honey, then top with the rest of the apples and some onion. Add powdered cinnamon to the top. This can be covered and cooked for eight hours.

3. Remove the apple and pork mixture and make sure you keep it warm. Move the juices from cooking over to a small pan, boiling it to reduce it. This can be served with the apple and pork mix and garnished with parsley.

As you can see, cooking doesn't have to be complicated. This book has given you a wide range of dishes, from very simple, to a bit more complex. Feel free to tackle them as soon as you're ready and add your own twists to them as you see fit! Good luck.

Conclusion

Thanks again for reading *Crock-pot Recipes: 60 Easy, Delicious, and Healthy Crock-pot Recipes for Busy People.* Hopefully, you now feel empowered and prepared to create your own delightful dishes at home using your handy Crock-pot.

You now know how to cook a suitable dish for any situation, whether it's a simple family dinner, a fancy party, a holiday, or your summer vacation. Impress your friends and family with your newfound abilities!

If you enjoyed this book, I'd like to ask you a favor. Please leave it a positive review on Amazon! Thank you and good luck.

Index

Recipe #21: Southwest Barley and Three Bean Soup.

Recipe #22: A Moroccan Lentil Crock-pot Dish.

Recipe #23: Red Curry Soup with Lentils.

Recipe #24: Traditional Pot Roast Dish.

Recipe #25: Fantastic Crock-pot Fajitas.

Recipe #26: Pork Roast Teriyaki.

Recipe #27: Delicious Slow Cooked Winter Stew.

Recipe #28: Onion and Apple Pot Roast.

Recipe #29: Crock-pot Stuffed Peppers.

Recipe #30: Pumpkin and Black Bean Chili.

Recipe #31: Italian Peppers and Chicken.

Recipe #32: Pineapple Mango Chicken Wraps.

Recipe #33: Super Green and Healthy Soup.

Recipe #34: Zesty Beef and Orange Dish.

Recipe #35: Couscous and Chicken dish.

Recipe #36: Crock-pot French Onion Soup.

Recipe #37: Crock-pot Berry and Turkey Compote.

Recipe #38: Crock-pot Pork Stew.

Recipe #39: Crock-pot Seafood Dish.

Recipe #40: Ham and Black-Eyed Peas.

Recipe #41: Veggie and Beef Dish.

www.ingramcontent.com/pod-product-compliance
Lightning Source LLC
Chambersburg PA
CBHW070811240726
48654CB00007B/300